WAYS TO STAY HEALTHY WHEN YOU WORK AT A DESK

TIPS FOR A HEALTHY LIFESTYLE

AHMED .R

Contents

CHAPTER ONE

INTRODUCTION

Many people find themselves spending a lot of time sitting at a desk in today's increasingly sedentary work conditions, which can be detrimental to their physical and emotional well-being. It is feasible to lead a healthy lifestyle while working at a desk, and it is crucial for general wellbeing. Your general health can be enhanced, stress can be decreased, and physical activity can be encouraged by implementing easy yet powerful tactics into your everyday routine. We'll look at useful advice and methods in this guide to keep you young and healthy when working at a desk. These tactics will enable you to put your health and well-being first at work, from implementing frequent activity breaks and ergonomic changes to encouraging good eating habits and stress management. One workstation at a time, let's set out on a journey to a more balanced, healthier existence.

The negative health effects of desk work

Long-term desk work has a number of negative health effects on one's physical and mental health. The following are some of the main health risks connected to desk work:

Sedentary Behavior: Extended periods of sitting have been connected to obesity, heart disease, and metabolic disorders, among other health problems. Desk workers frequently spend long hours sitting down, which raises health hazards and lowers levels of physical activity.

Musculoskeletal Issues: Repetitive motions and poor posture can result in carpal tunnel syndrome, neck and back pain, and repetitive strain injuries (RSIs). These problems are exacerbated by poor ergonomics and extended sitting, which lead to discomfort and decreased productivity.

Obesity and Weight Gain: Excessive sedentary behavior and a lack of physical activity can lead to obesity and weight gain. Because desk workers have less opportunities for activity and calorie expenditure during the day, they may be more susceptible to weight-related health issues.

Eye strain and other vision issues can result from prolonged computer screen staring. Other symptoms include dry eyes and eye strain. Inadequate screen settings, glare, and bad lighting all make this worse, which impairs vision and causes discomfort.

Desk employment can also have an adverse effect on mental health, increasing the risk of stress, anxiety, and depression. Tight deadlines, heavy workloads, and a poor work-life balance all contribute to these problems, which have an adverse effect on productivity and general well-being.

Bad Eating Habits: Working at a desk might encourage bad eating habits like skipping meals, consuming sugary drinks, and snacking on processed foods. Both physical and mental health can be negatively impacted by poor diet, which can cause weight gain, exhaustion, and low energy levels.

Decreased Physical Fitness: Decreased physical fitness and general health might result from a lack of opportunity for physical activity throughout the workday. The risk of chronic diseases and other health issues is increased for desk workers who may find it difficult to maintain prescribed activity levels.

Social Isolation: Extended periods of time spent seated at a desk might result in a decline in social interaction and social isolation. Insufficient possibilities for in-person interaction and communication can have an adverse effect on an individual's mental health and level of job satisfaction.

weariness and Sleep disruptions: Prolonged screen usage and sedentary activity can cause sleep disruptions and weariness by interfering with sleep rhythms. Inadequate sleep has an adverse effect on mood, cognition, and general health, which in turn impairs productivity at work and quality of life.

Increased Risk of Chronic Disease: Chronic diseases like obesity, diabetes, heart disease, and some types of cancer are more likely to occur as a result of sedentary activity, poor posture, and unhealthy lifestyle choices.

It takes proactive steps to support physical activity, enhance ergonomics, give mental health first priority, and cultivate healthy living habits in order to address these health issues. People can improve their health and well-being at work by implementing techniques to lessen the negative impacts of desk labor.

The significance of preserving health in spite of sedentary occupations

It's important to maintain your health even if you work sedentary jobs for the reasons listed below:

Decreased Risk of Chronic Illnesses: Being physically active on a regular basis helps to ward off chronic illnesses like diabetes, obesity, heart disease, and some cancers. Making physical activity a priority can help reduce these hazards and support long-term health even in the case of a sedentary employment.

Enhanced Mental Health: Research has demonstrated that engaging in physical activity can significantly improve mental health, including lowering levels of stress, anxiety, and sadness. Including exercise and movement breaks in your job can improve your mood, sharpen your mind, and make you feel better overall.

Increased Physical Fitness: Muscle strength and physical fitness are frequently impacted by sedentary work responsibilities. Maintaining physical fitness, strength, and flexibility through regular exercise and daily movement can lower the risk of musculoskeletal issues and increase total functional capability.

Improved Posture and Ergonomics: Extended desk sitting can cause musculoskeletal problems such neck strain, back discomfort, and repetitive strain injuries in addition to poor posture. Incorporating standing or walking into the work routine, taking pauses for stretching, and following good ergonomics can all help reduce these issues and preserve spinal health.

Enhanced Productivity and Energy: Research indicates that engaging in regular physical activity might boost one's energy levels, concentration, and cognitive abilities. Despite having a sedentary work, people can improve their overall job performance, creativity, and productivity by remaining active.

Enhanced Immune Function: Being inactive and sedentary can impair immunity, making a person more vulnerable to diseases and illnesses. Frequent exercise strengthens the immune system, lowering the risk of disease and enhancing the body's natural defenses.

Benefits for Longevity: Regular physical activity is linked to a longer lifespan and better quality of life for senior citizens. Even with a sedentary work, leading an active lifestyle lowers the incidence of chronic illnesses and preserves functional independence, which can promote lifespan and healthy aging.

Better Sleep: Getting regular exercise helps people sleep for longer periods of time and with higher quality, both of which are critical for general health and wellbeing. Despite the pressures of a sedentary work schedule, making exercise a priority and sticking to a regular sleep schedule can assist improve sleep quality and general health.

Preventing chronic diseases, fostering mental health, boosting physical fitness, and raising general quality of life all depend on keeping health despite sedentary employment duties. Through the implementation of appropriate ergonomic practices, emphasizing physical activity, and embracing healthy lifestyle choices, individuals can effectively address the negative consequences of sedentary employment and ultimately enhance their overall health and well-being.

An Ergonomic Configuration

Setting up an ergonomic workspace is crucial to preserving health and wellbeing when using a desk job. The following are essential elements of an ergonomic workstation:

Chair: Select a chair that helps you maintain proper posture and supports your lower back. Seek for a chair with armrests, lumbar support, and height adjustment. Make sure your thighs are parallel to the floor and your feet are flat on the floor or supported by a footrest.

Desk: Choose a desk that will enable you to access your computer and other equipment with ease and to keep good posture. When typing, your elbows should be 90 degrees bent, your wrists should be straight, and your shoulders should be relaxed, depending on the height of your workstation.

Placement of the Monitor: To ease the pressure on your neck and upper back, place the monitor at eye level. The monitor should be an arm's length away from your body, with the top of the screen at or slightly below eye level.

Keyboard and Mouse: Straighten your wrists and keep your elbows close to your body while you position the keyboard and mouse within easy reach. When typing and using the mouse, keep your wrists in a neutral position by using a wrist rest.

Monitor Distance: To lessen eye strain, hold your monitor arm's length away from your body. To reduce glare and reflection, adjust the brightness and contrast settings. You should also take regular pauses to give your eyes a chance to rest.

Keyboard Tray: To reduce keyboard height and free up work space, think about utilizing a keyboard tray. This lessens the chance of repetitive strain injuries and helps preserve good alignment of the wrists and arms.

Document Holder: To lessen neck strain and increase productivity, use a document holder that is the same height and distance from your monitor if you regularly consult documents while typing.

Lighting: To lessen eye strain and fatigue, make sure your office is well-lit. To reduce glare on your computer screen and brighten the space around your workstation, use task lighting.

Footrest: To support your feet and keep good posture when seated, use a footrest if your feet are not touching the floor. This encourages blood flow in your legs and relieves pressure on your lower back.

Regular Breaks: Throughout the day, take regular pauses to stretch, stand up, and move around. Make a note to take a brief break every hour to avoid being stiff and lower your chance of developing musculoskeletal issues.

By putting these ergonomic guidelines into practice and designing a cozy workstation, you may lower your risk of weariness, pain, and accidents when working at a desk and enhance your long-term health and wellbeing.

Frequent Rest Periods

You may counteract the negative effects of extended sitting and promote health and well-being while working at a desk by including regular exercise breaks into your daily routine.

CHAPTER TWO

The following advice will help you fit in activity breaks throughout your workday:

Plan Your Breaks: Make a note of when to take breaks throughout the day by setting alarms or reminders. Every hour, try to take a quick break to get up, stretch, and walk around.

Stretching Exercises: To reduce muscle tension and increase flexibility, use basic stretching exercises. To offset the affects of prolonged sitting, concentrate on stretching your legs, hips, shoulders, back, and neck.

Desk Exercises: Work out at your desk to strengthen your muscles and improve blood circulation. Calf raises, desk push-ups, chair squats, and sitting leg lifts are a few examples. You may perform these workouts covertly and without getting up from your desk.

Walk Breaks: During your breaks, take quick strolls outside or around the workplace. A quick stroll can increase energy, lessen stiffness, and promote better circulation. To add more exercise to your day, wherever possible, take the stairs rather than the elevator.

Stand-Up Desk: To switch between sitting and standing during the day, think about utilizing an adjustable desk converter or standing desk. In addition to improving posture, standing short periods of time can assist lower the health hazards connected with extended sitting.

Active Commuting: Try to walk, cycle, or take public transportation as a way to fit in some exercise during your daily commute. This raises your level of general activity by enabling you to exercise at the beginning and conclusion of your workday.

Microbreaks: Take quick, regular breaks to move about, stretch, and stand up. Every 30 minutes, even a one- to two-minute rest can help prevent soreness and lessen muscular fatigue.

Breathing Techniques: To lower tension, improve oxygen flow, and encourage relaxation, engage in deep breathing techniques. For a short while, concentrate on your breathing, taking slow, deep breaths through your nose and releasing them through your mouth.

Active Meetings: Consider holding standing or walking conversations during meetings as an alternative to sitting down. This enhances concentration and productivity while promoting movement, creativity, and teamwork.

Water intervals: Take use of the chance to get up, stretch, and move about during hydration intervals. In order to stay hydrated and support general health, sip water frequently throughout the day.

You may lessen the negative consequences of sedentary behavior, boost energy levels, increase productivity, and promote general health and well-being by implementing these regular activity breaks into your workplace. Try out a variety of tactics to see which one suits you the most, and incorporate activity into your everyday routine as naturally as possible.

Stretching Activities

You may offset the effects of extended sitting and maintain flexibility, posture, and general well-being while working at a desk by including stretching activities into your daily routine. The following are some efficient stretches created especially for desk workers:

Neck Stretch: Take a tall seat on your chair and tilt your head slightly to one side. Press your ear to your shoulder until you feel your neck getting stretched out. After holding for 15 to 30 seconds, swap sides. By gently nodding your head forward and backward, you can also execute a forward and backward neck stretch.

Shoulder stretches involve putting your fingers together and extending your arms above with your palms facing up. Lean forward, expanding your chest and extending your spine toward the ceiling. Release after holding for 15 to 30 seconds. Shaking your shoulders up towards your ears, rolling them back, and then down in a circular motion is another way to conduct shoulder rolls.

Stretch your upper back by sitting up straight and putting your hands together in front of you with the palms facing out. Feel a stretch between your shoulder blades as you round your back and push your hands away from your body. Release after holding for 15 to 30 seconds.

Chest Opener: Squeeze your shoulder blades together while sitting or standing erect and clasping your hands behind your back. Feel a stretch across the front of your shoulders and chest as you slightly raise your arms and open your chest. Release after holding for 15 to 30 seconds.

Seated Spinal Twist: Raise your seat to a sitting position and rest your right hand on the chair's back. With your left hand supporting your right leg while you twist your torso to the right, do so. Turn your upper body slightly and cast your gaze over your right shoulder. After holding for 15 to 30 seconds, swap sides.

Seated Hip Stretch: Keep your right foot flexed to protect your knee as you sit closer to the front of the chair and cross your right ankle across your left knee. You should feel a stretch in your right hip and glute as you sit up straight and bend forward at the hips. After holding for 15 to 30 seconds, swap sides.

Stretch your hamstrings by sitting on the edge of your chair and extending your right leg forward with your toes pointed upward and your heel on the floor. Hinge forward at the hips while maintaining a straight back until you feel your right leg stretching. After holding for 15 to 30 seconds, swap sides.

Calf Stretch: Using a desk or wall as support, stand up and place your hands there. Reposition your right foot while maintaining a straight stride and firmly planting your heel on the ground. Feel the stretch in your right calf as you slant forward and gently bend your left knee. After holding for 15 to 30 seconds, swap sides.

Regularly engage in these stretches throughout the day to ease tense muscles, enhance blood flow, and encourage good posture and flexibility. Never forget to take deep breaths and go slowly with each stretch, without making any quick or jerky motions. Including stretching breaks in your workday can help reduce soreness, boost vitality, and improve general health.

Appropriate Posture Awareness

When working at a desk, maintaining good posture is crucial for avoiding musculoskeletal problems and enhancing general health and wellbeing. Here are some pointers to help you stay mindful of your posture:

Straighten Your Back: Lean back in your chair and press your back into the backrest. Avoid slouching or slumping forward; instead, maintain a straight spine and relaxed shoulders.

Head and Neck Alignment: Maintain a straight head-over-spine alignment by avoiding excessive forward or backward tilting. Your chin should be parallel to the floor and your ears should be in line with your shoulders.

Chair Height Adjustment: Set your chair height such that your knees are at a 90-degree angle and your feet are flat on the ground or supported by a footrest. Your hips should be just above your knees, and your thighs should be parallel to the floor.

Arrange Your Keyboard and Mouse: Hold your elbows close to your body and your wrists straight when you place your keyboard and mouse at elbow level. To save reaching and straining, keep your mouse and keyboard close at hand.

Employ the Correct Monitor Positioning: Hold your monitor arm's length in front of you, with the top of the screen at or just below eye level.

To lessen eye strain and neck strain, change the monitor's height and angle.

Take Regular Breaks: Throughout the day, take brief pauses to stand up, stretch, and adjust your posture. Make it a habit to get up, stretch, or take a stroll every hour to avoid becoming stiff and lower your chance of developing musculoskeletal issues.

Use Your Core: To support your spine and keep your stability while sitting, use your abdominal muscles. Bring your navel gently up towards your spine to prevent slouching or arching your lower back.

Employ Good Ergonomics: Make sure your workstation is arranged ergonomically to encourage good posture and lessen strain. If required, use an ergonomic chair, a supportive cushion, or a chair with lumbar support.

Practice Posture Checks: Throughout the day, make sure you are sitting or standing properly by periodically checking your posture. If necessary, use mirrors or ask a coworker to give you comments on your posture.

Remain Aware of Your Posture: When working, be aware of your posture. Make an effort to sit or stand up straight and keep your body in the right alignment. Maintain proper posture by not hunching forward or slouching, and by making changes as necessary.

You may improve general comfort and well-being when working at a desk, support spinal health, and lower your risk of musculoskeletal problems by paying attention to your posture and incorporating these suggestions into your daily routine. Maintaining good posture awareness on a regular basis can boost one's vitality, productivity, and long-term health.

Optimal Snacking Practices

Sustaining energy levels, focus, and general well-being when working at a desk requires maintaining appropriate snacking habits. The following advice will help you fit in some nutritious snacks during the workday:

Plan Ahead: Make the time to organize and prepare wholesome snacks ahead of time so that you will always have wholesome options on hand for when hunger pangs come. To keep at your desk or in the office refrigerator, stock up on fresh fruits, veggies, nuts, seeds, yogurt, and other healthful snacks.

Select Nutrient-Rich Foods: Make sure your snacks are high in vitamins, minerals, fiber, protein, and healthy fats. To keep you feeling full and energized, choose whole foods over processed snacks and try to incorporate a balance of carbs, protein, and healthy fats.

Portion Control: To prevent overindulging and ingesting too many calories when snacking, exercise portion control. To divide out your snacks, use tiny bowls or containers rather than just mindlessly eating them right out of the bag or packet.

Remain Hydrated: Keep a bottle of water on your desk and drink plenty of water throughout the day. As dehydration can occasionally be confused with hunger, staying hydrated and reducing cravings will help you feel satisfied in between meals.

including Protein: To assist sustain energy levels and encourage satiety, including protein-rich snacks in your daily diet. Lean meats or chicken, hard-boiled eggs, hummus with vegetables, Greek yogurt, and nuts and seeds are a few examples.

Add Fiber: To aid with digestion, control blood sugar, and encourage feelings of fullness, select snacks that are high in fiber. Fruits, vegetables, whole grains, nuts, seeds, and legumes are examples of foods high in fiber.

Restrict Added Sugars and Processed Foods: Restrict added sugars, processed carbs, and unhealthy fats in your snacking because they can cause energy dumps and cravings. Rather, choose complete, minimally processed foods that offer long-lasting energy and health advantages.

Snack Intentionally: Give your snacks some thought and take some time to appreciate their flavor, texture, and satisfaction. Eat with attention on fueling your body and sating your appetite, not on work or devices.

Be Ready for Cravings: Stock up on nutritious food to quell cravings and stop yourself from grabbing bad ones on the spur of the moment. Selecting snacks you look forward to and enjoy will help you avoid temptation and make healthier decisions.

Listen to Your Body: Rather than snacking out of boredom or habit, pay attention to your body's signals of hunger and fullness. Eat carefully and gently, ending when you're content rather than feeling stuffed.

While working at a desk, you may maintain your energy levels, focus, and general health by adopting these wholesome eating practices. You can maintain your energy, concentration, and productivity throughout the day by making thoughtful food choices and selecting nutrient-rich snacks.

Drinking Water

Maintaining good health and well-being requires drinking enough of water, especially when working long hours at a desk. The following advice will help you stay hydrated when working at a desk:

Drink A Lot of Water: Even if you don't feel thirsty, try to stay hydrated by drinking water frequently throughout the day. To stay hydrated, keep a bottle of water at your desk and take periodic sips. To help you remain on track, set a goal for yourself to drink a specified amount of water by a specific time each day.

Employ a Hydration Reminder: Utilize your computer or phone to set up reminders to remember you to sip water on a regular basis. Reminder-equipped smart water bottles and apps can also help you remember to drink enough water throughout the day and keep yourself accountable.

Naturally Flavor Water: If you think plain water is boring, consider adding tastes like lemon, cucumber, mint, or berries. You may enjoy drinking water more and be more inclined to drink it throughout the day by adding a dash of flavor.

Keep an Eye on the Color of Your Urine: Your urine's color might serve as a straightforward sign of your level of hydration. Urine that is straw-colored or pale yellow in color shows that you are well hydrated. Dehydration and the need to consume more water may be indicated by darker urine.

Limit Sugary and Caffeinated Drinks: Although occasionally indulging in sugary or caffeinated drinks is acceptable, keep in mind how they affect hydration. When ingested in excess, caffeine and sugar have the potential to cause dehydration as they function as diuretics, increasing the production of urine.

Consume Hydrating Foods: To enhance your water intake, include hydrating foods in your meals and snacks. High-water fruits and vegetables, such watermelon, cucumbers, strawberries, oranges, and celery, can support your general levels of hydration.

Keep an eye on the air quality because dry indoor air, particularly in climate-controlled office settings, can lead to dehydration. If you live in a dry area especially during the winter, think about using a humidifier to provide moisture into the air and keep people from becoming dehydrated.

Hydrate Before, During, and After Exercise: Make sure you drink enough water before, during, and after any physical activity you do during breaks or after work. To stay hydrated and aid in recovery, sip water prior to exercise, rehydrate subsequently, and drink more water afterward.

Listen to Your Body: When you feel thirsty, follow your body's instructions and sip water. Don't ignore your thirst; it's your body's way of telling you that it needs water.

Monitor Your Water Intake: Use a notebook, an app, or other water tracking tool to keep track of how much water you drink each day. You can make sure you're meeting your hydration goals and maintain accountability by keeping an eye on how much water you're consuming.

You can maintain your general health, energy levels, focus, and productivity while working at a desk by paying attention to your water needs and implementing these suggestions throughout your workday. Make it a practice to drink water on a regular basis to stay hydrated, as this is crucial for both good performance and overall health.

Techniques for Stress Management

Maintaining general health and wellbeing requires effective stress management, particularly when working long hours at a desk. The following stress-reduction methods can help you maintain your health while working at a desk:

Deep Breathing Exercises: To relax the body and soothe the mind, engage in deep breathing exercises. Breathe in slowly and deeply through your nose to fill your lungs, and out slowly through your mouth.

CHAPTER THREE

Repeat this sequence multiple times, paying attention to each breath and letting go of tension with each exhale.

Mindfulness Meditation: To develop awareness and lower stress, incorporate mindfulness meditation into your everyday practice. Spend a few minutes every day in silence, concentrating on your breathing, your body's feelings, or the here and now without passing judgment. You can learn to meditate with mindfulness to become more robust and grounded when dealing with stress.

Progressive Muscle Relaxation: To ease physical stress and encourage relaxation, practice progressive muscle relaxation. Work your way up to your head and neck by methodically tensing and relaxing each muscle group in your body, starting from your toes. With every muscle area you relax, concentrate on letting go of stress and releasing tension.

Stress-Busting Desk Exercises: To relieve stress and improve circulation, including desk exercises in your daily routine. Easy yoga poses, chair exercises, or stretches can help ease physical pain and lower stress levels all day long.

Plan Regular Breaks: Allocate time each day for rest and rejuvenation. During your break, get up from your desk, stretch, take a quick stroll, or do something fun and relaxing for yourself. By taking pauses, you can avoid burnout and come back to your work with fresh enthusiasm and focus.

Set Boundaries: To stop stress from leaking into other aspects of your life, clearly define boundaries between your personal and professional lives. Establish clear work schedules, allot time for rest periods and breaks, and give priority to self-care pursuits after work.

Practice Time Management: Make use of time management strategies to avoid feeling overburdened by your workload, prioritize your duties, and set reasonable deadlines. To lower stress and boost productivity, divide big jobs into smaller, more doable tasks and take them one step at a time.

Seek Social Support: Make connections with family, friends, or coworkers to get company and social support. During trying times, having a support system can help you share experiences, manage stress, and gain perspective.

Develop an Attitude of Gratitude: Make a daily list of the things for which you are thankful. Maintaining a gratitude diary, expressing gratitude to others, or just pausing to acknowledge the good things in your life can help you deflect stress and foster wellbeing.

Seek Professional Assistance if Needed: Don't be afraid to ask for help from a mental health professional if you're finding it difficult to manage your stress on your own. Stress management programs, therapy, and counseling can offer helpful coping mechanisms and techniques to help you feel better overall.

While working at a desk, you can effectively manage stress, foster mental and emotional resilience, and preserve general health and well-being by implementing these stress management practices into your daily routine. Recall that stress management is a lifetime process, and it could take some trial and error and self-discovery to figure out what suits you best.

Eye Health

When working at a desk, especially if you spend a lot of time in front of a computer screen, it's imperative to take care of your eyes. The following eye care advice may help you maintain your health when working at a desk:

Observe the 20-20-20 Rule: Every 20 minutes, take a 20-second break and stare at something at least 20 feet away to reduce eye strain. By doing this, the eye strain and weariness brought on by extended screen time are lessened.

Modify Monitor Settings: To cut down on glare and improve legibility, change the font size, brightness, and contrast on your computer screen. To reduce eye strain, place your monitor at arm's length from your eyes and at eye level.

Blink Often: When working at a desk, it's important to remember to blink frequently because prolonged screen looking can lower blink rates and cause dry eyes. Blinking relieves dryness and irritation by rehydrating and moisturizing the eyes.

Employ Appropriate Lighting: To lessen eye strain, make sure your workspace is well-lit. When feasible, use natural or indirect lighting. To reduce glare from windows or overhead lights, adjust your curtains or use a glare filter on your computer.

Take Regular rests: To minimize eye tiredness and to relax your eyes, take regular rests in addition to adhering to the 20-20-20 rule. Occasionally take a break from your screen, stand up, stretch, and allow your eyes to rest and heal.

Use Computer Eyewear: To lessen eye strain and shield your eyes from the damaging effects of blue light released by digital screens, think about using computer glasses or blue light-blocking glasses. By minimizing glare and blocking out blue light, these glasses can lessen eye strain and increase comfort.

Keep Your Eyes Moist: If you suffer from dryness or irritation in your eyes when working at a desk, use artificial tears or lubricating eye drops to keep your eyes pleasant and moist. Utilize the drops as needed throughout the day, according to the directions on the product packaging.

Use Good Ergonomics: To lessen neck and eye strain, use good ergonomics when working at a desk. To make sure that your eyes are straight ahead and centered on the top of the screen, adjust the height and distance of your chair, keyboard, and monitor.

Keep Yourself Hydrated: To stay hydrated and sustain ideal tear production, sip on lots of water throughout the day. Make sure you consume enough water to keep your body and eyes hydrated because dehydration can aggravate eye strain and cause dry eyes.

Get Regular Eye Exams: To keep an eye on the health of your eyes and to address any visual issues or conditions, make an appointment for routine eye exams with an optometrist or ophthalmologist. Frequent examinations can help keep your eyes healthy while working at a desk by identifying problems early on.

You can safeguard your eyes and keep your eyes in optimal condition while working at a desk by implementing these eye care tips into your daily routine. To ensure that you can continue to work comfortably and effectively for years to come, always remember to prioritize the health of your eyes and take preventative measures to avoid eye strain and discomfort.

Social Interaction

Keeping up social ties is essential for general health and wellbeing, particularly for those who work at desks where sedentary behavior and isolation are commonplace. Here are a few strategies for maintaining social connections while seated at a desk:

Plan Social Breaks: Schedule time during your workday to engage in face-to-face or virtual conversations with colleagues. Take time during breaks to chat, exchange ideas, or just establish a personal connection.

Join Clubs or Workplace organizations: Take part in social committees, clubs, or workplace organizations to network and participate in common interests. Participating in volunteer work, attending reading clubs, or wellness initiatives can offer chances for networking and community service.

Take Lunch Breaks with Others: Arrange group meals or activities, or simply request coworkers to join you for lunch rather than dining alone at your desk. Mealtime ties are strengthened and camaraderie is fostered, which improves social connections at work.

Attend Social Events: Make the most of the get-togethers your workplace hosts, like Christmas parties, happy hours, and team-building exercises. By taking part in these activities, you can strengthen your relationships and socialize with coworkers outside of the office.

Utilize Communication Tools: Keep in touch with colleagues by making use of collaboration platforms, video conferencing software, and instant messaging. Throughout the day, use these tools to converse casually, exchange updates, and pose inquiries.

Reach Out to Remote Colleagues: Try to stay in touch and establish frequent connections with colleagues who operate remotely or off-site. Plan online video conferences, team meetings, or coffee dates to stay in touch and feel like you belong.

Take Part in Networking Events: To grow your professional network and meet new people, go to conferences, industry meetups, or networking events. By connecting with experts from various industries and backgrounds, networking creates new potential for partnerships and relationships.

Remain Involved on Social Media: Make use of social media channels to maintain relationships with colleagues, colleagues in the field, and professional contacts. To keep in touch and learn about their whereabouts, follow coworkers on social media sites like Twitter, LinkedIn, and Instagram and reply to their posts.

Ask for Help: Don't be afraid to ask for help from friends, family, or coworkers if you're feeling anxious, overwhelmed, or alone. Seeking out social support and expressing your emotions can reduce stress and enhance general wellbeing.

Set a positive example for others by taking initiative to promote an inclusive and socially connected work environment. Start discussions, extend invitations to social events, and provide chances for cooperation and partnership.

Whether you work at a desk, you may improve your general health and well-being, lessen feelings of loneliness, and strengthen your sense of belonging by making social relationships a priority and actively searching out opportunities to connect with others. Keep in mind that while establishing and sustaining connections is work, the advantages of social interaction are priceless.

Summary

In summary, maintaining physical, mental, and social well-being while working at a desk necessitates a multimodal strategy. Despite the drawbacks of a sedentary workplace, you can retain your best level of productivity and health by implementing a number of measures into your everyday routine.

There are several ways to maintain your health when working at a desk, from proper setup and frequent activity breaks to stress reduction methods and wholesome eating habits. Common problems including musculoskeletal disorders, eye strain, stress, and isolation can be avoided by placing a high priority on good posture, hydration, eye care, and social interaction.

Throughout the workday, it's critical to pay attention to your body, take breaks when necessary, and engage in self-care in order to preserve equilibrium and wellbeing. You may stay healthy and vibrant for the long term while thriving in your desk-based employment by implementing healthy behaviors, reaching out for social support, and creating a happy work environment.

To support your health and well-being when working at a desk, start putting these suggestions into practice right away. Keep in mind that little changes can have a large impact. You may maximize your performance, happiness, and quality of life at work and in other areas of your life by taking a holistic approach to health and self-care.

THE END

www.ingramcontent.com/pod-product-compliance
Lightning Source LLC
Chambersburg PA
CBHW051919250726

48659CB00002B/736